PALEO BEGINNERS

The "Eat Like a Caveman" Paleo Diet Fast Track Guide to Better Health and Vitality

Including a 7-Day Meal Plan and Delicious Paleo Recipes

Gina Crawford

Copyright © 2014 by Gina Crawford

All rights reserved. No part of this publication may be reproduced, distributed, or transmitted in any form or by any means, including photocopying, recording, or other electronic or mechanical methods without the prior written permission of the publisher, except in the case of brief quotations embodied in critical reviews and certain other non-commercial uses permitted by copyright law. For permission, direct requests to the publisher. Distribution of this book without the prior permission of the author is illegal and therefore punishable by law.

Evita Publishing, PO Box 306, Station A, Vancouver Island, BC V9W 5B1 Canada

IMPORTANT

The information in this book reflects the author's experience, research, and opinions and is not intended to replace medical advice.

Before beginning this or any nutritional or exercise regimen, consult your physician to be sure it is appropriate for you. Ask for a physical stress test.

Table of Contents

Introduction 6

Chapter 1

What is the Paleo Diet? 9

Chapter 2

What You Can and Can't Eat on the Paleo Diet? 20

Chapter 3

Why Go Paleo? 25

Chapter 4

How the Paleo Diet Compares? .41

Chapter 5

How the Paleo Diet is Your Body's Best Friend 46

Chapter 6

7-Day Meal Plan and Recipes .54

Chapter 7

Tips for Sticking with the Paleo Diet 93

Conclusion 96

Introduction

Congratulations for being proactive about improving or maintaining the quality of your health to purchase the book *"Paleo for Beginners: The "Eat Like a Caveman" FAST TRACK GUIDE to Better Health and Vitality, Including a 7-Day Meal Plan and Delicious Paleo Recipes."*

Let's face it, you're busy, yet you want to know the best, most effective way to nurture your health long term. This book has been designed with you in mind. It is a no-fluff, to-the-point quick read that is jam-packed with the necessary information you need to achieve better health and vitality by applying the Paleo diet to your life.

In this book you will learn the essentials of the Paleo diet: how to choose foods that allow your body to function at its best, how foods work inside your body to either help or hurt you, why eating foods in their most natural state is important, what you can and can't eat on a Paleo diet, what a Paleo meal looks like, how to lose weight on the Paleo diet and much more.

As an added bonus, this book also includes Paleo breakfast, lunch, dinner and snack recipes. There is a 7-day meal plan included as well that will allow you to dive right into super-charged, healthy eating.

Congratulations again for taking your health into your own hands by purchasing this book!

Chapter 1

What is the Paleo Diet?

"Let food be thy medicine and medicine be thy food."
Hippocrates

The Paleolithic diet or Paleo diet is also called the caveman diet or the Stone Age diet because it is based on the consumption of plants and animals that were eaten during the Paleolithic era. Proponents of this diet believe that if we apply the eating habits of the Paleolithic people to our lives, we will decrease the likelihood of acquiring disease through food.

History

The modern Paleo diet was invented by Walter Voegtlin, a gastroenterologist and author who published his findings about the diet in his book, *The Stone Age Diet*, in 1975. He studied Paleolithic eating habits in an effort to find a cure for Crohn's disease, colitis, irritable bowel syndrome and indigestion. He believed that the early human diet could affect these conditions in a positive way and improve them significantly without side effects.

Voegtlin took a particular interest in the carnivorous side of humans. He asserted that humans were meant to eat protein and fat primarily found in meat. Carbohydrates were only to be consumed in small amounts whereas fresh fruits and vegetables were to be consumed in larger amounts on a daily basis.

Thirteen years after Voegtlin introduced the concept of the Paleo diet, Konner, Eaton and Shostak wrote a book about the diet with a twist. They focused on eating the same portions of fats, proteins and carbohydrates as in the Paleolithic era rather than excluding foods from the diet. Their version of the diet allowed the consumption of brown rice, potatoes and whole grain bread as well as skim milk and other dairy products which were not allowed in Voegtlin's version of the Paleo diet. Their reason for including these foods was because it wasn't the individual food that made the Paleo eating habits healthy but rather the proportions of nutrients in those foods.

The Paleo diet originated from the human's instinctive need to survive in the harshest conditions known in human history. This diet is being revived by athletes and dieters who strongly believe that it has stood the test of time and offers just the right balance of nutrients needed for health and physical performance.

Theory behind the Paleo diet

It is strongly believed that the Paleo diet is still effective today because of the way that the modern genetic code has evolved. 99.9% of human genetics have been the same for the past 10,000 years. The body uses food the same way it did back in the

Paleolithic era, and while the environment has changed, the physical body has not.

The 'fight or flight' response was essential to the early humans. Almost all of their activities involved strenuous physical activity because they had to rely on hunting and gathering food to survive. The high level of activity kept them in shape and enabled their bodies to process the food they ate efficiently.

The plants the Paleolithic people ate grew naturally and had no chemicals in them. They also consumed lower measures of carbohydrates in each meal. Because the glycemic load of their meals was low, the food had less negative impact on the body's blood insulin level.

Mans modern diet differs from this in that it contains overly processed starches and sugars. This has a negative impact on the body. Early humans were able to eat and convert their food to energy without having any alarming blood sugar effects. Modern mans more sedentary lifestyle paired with the consumption of processed foods and carbohydrates causes higher blood insulin levels and weight gain.

Studies have shown that when early Paleolithic humans started eating lean meat, their brains and bodies started to develop rapidly. The animals that they hunted were wild, and did not have excess fat in them to cause heart ailments. The Paleo diet therefore encourages eating only grass-fed meat as opposed to grain fed. It also highly encourages the consumption of bison and wild game over beef and farmed animals.

Some modern-day cultures that still live in a hunter-gatherer society are thriving. These cultures are living proof of the benefits of this diet. Furthermore, the main belief of the Paleo diet is that if humans were to adapt the Paleolithic diet to their lives, there would be a significant decrease in heart disease, obesity and diabetes. The Paleo diet functions on the belief that modern food processing has caused many of today's diseases. Therefore, if we return to a simpler, more natural, unprocessed way of eating we will see a significant decrease in disease and a rise in sustainable health.

Paleo diet basics

Though there are varied versions of the Paleo diet, scientists and nutritionists agree on the following underlying principles that support the effectiveness of the diet:

Eat like a caveman

Eat what the early humans ate. Our bodies were designed to function best on natural foods of the land. The more we choose to eat foods in their most natural state, the healthier we will be.

Eat organic or wild meat

Organically raised animals are the only source of meat acceptable on the Paleo diet. Wild grass-fed animals like deer or buffalo are preferred over domesticated cattle because they are leaner meats and closer to what Paleolithic people would have eaten. Fish and seafood are also included in the Paleo diet as a great source of protein and healthy omega-3s.

Eat all kinds of fruits and vegetables

All kinds of fruits are allowed on the Paleo diet except those that are sugared or dried. Consuming whole fruits rather than fruit juices is more nutritious and a lower calorie choice, so choose whole fruits. Also, eating lots of vegetables, root crops and watery vegetables is highly encouraged because the fiber in plant-based foods replaces carbohydrates that you would normally get from grains. Fruits and vegetables also contain numerous vitamins that are essential to good health.

Say no to processed foods

Foods like chips, cookies and processed foods didn't exist during the Paleolithic era. Processed foods contain additives and chemicals that are harmful to your health. Exclude refined sugars and processed foods and choose foods that are free from preservatives and flavorings. This will reduce your sodium intake and calories. The key is to choose food that has not been altered from its simplest, most basic form.

Get rid of table salt

Salt is not necessary when eating fresh food. Meat has natural salt in it so adding more salt can cause high blood pressure and an imbalance of electrolytes.

Cooking is okay

Though the Paleo diet encourages eating organic raw foods, it recognizes that cavemen did cook their food as well. Cooking is perfectly acceptable as long as you are also eating several servings of raw fruits and vegetables daily.

Chapter 2

What You Can and Can't Eat on the Paleo Diet?

Eat :o)

Grass-fed meats

Fish/seafood

Eggs

Fruits/Vegetables

Healthy oils

Nuts and seeds

Sweet potatoes

Note: Vegetables with a high starch content such as regular potatoes and squash have low nutritional value compared to the amount of carbohydrates, sugars and starch you get from eating them. There is some debate over consuming starchy vegetables on the Paleo diet. They are high on the glycemic index scale which can affect blood sugar levels in a negative way.

Potatoes and the Paleo diet: Loren Cordain in his book "The Paleo Diet" said that it was fine to eat sweet potatoes in moderation but to avoid regular potatoes. Regular potatoes contain anti-nutrients like saponins that are not good for you. Sweet potatoes are free from saponins and therefore a healthier choice.

Don't Eat :o(

Processed foods

Refined sugar

Salt

Legumes (including peanuts)

Dairy

Grains

Refined vegetable oils

Regular potatoes

Note: Peanuts are a legume, not a nut. They contain lectins and phytic acid which can cause inflammation and gastrointestinal pain. They also contain additives and a high level of salt.

What a Paleo meal looks like

Aim at eating 3-4 meals per day with protein as part of every meal. The majority of your meals should include the following: 4-8 oz of lean protein like chicken, turkey, pork loin, lean beef or seafood along with several servings of raw, steamed or lightly cooked vegetables. Eggs are also an excellent source of protein that should be included in your diet.

Top off each meal with good fats like walnut, coconut, or avocado oil. A handful of unsalted nuts like cashews, pecans, macadamias, almonds, walnuts or hazelnuts are also a great way of getting the good fats your body needs. Also include seeds like sunflower, flax and pumpkin seeds in your diet. Seeds double as a great source of good fat and protein.

Limit fruit consumption to one serving if your goal is to lose weight. Also limit nuts to 1-2 oz to lose weight. Beverages can include unsweetened tea, coffee (black) or water. No artificial sweeteners are allowed. Even Stevia should be avoided.

Chapter 3
Why Go Paleo?

The Paleo diet has been receiving worldwide attention because of its claim to improve our overall health. There are several benefits associated with the caveman diet. Some of them include:

Weight loss

One of the reasons that the Paleo diet is effective in weight loss is that it doesn't allow refined sugar. Foods that are high in calories such as candy, potato chips and cookies are often low in nutrients, especially if they are made with refined flour. If these carbohydrates are not converted to energy right away, they are stored in the body as fat.

Sweets can also have a negative effect on blood sugar making it spike and then crash. Fluctuating insulin levels and cortisol spikes eventually contribute to weight gain. Because the Paleo diet eliminates refined sugar and grains and introduces quality protein, it builds muscles and balances out sugar levels. Healthy fats are used by the body as a source of energy. Fruits and vegetables provide several nutrients and fibre that are essential to good health.

The Paleo diet gets rid of excess weight due to water retention. When the body consumes carbohydrates, the cells hold on to the excess water that the carbohydrates carry. This was a useful bodily function for the Paleolithic people because it enabled them to do sustained physical work without needing much water. In today's sedentary society however, the excess water that comes from eating too many carbohydrates in the form of grains, sugar and legumes soon turns into excess weight when glucose stores are used up and the extra water is released into the body. When people first go on the Paleo diet they experience increased thirst and more trips to the bathroom to release the stored excess water. As they release water from their body they begin to lose weight.

Gluten is something that a lot of people are sensitive to. Gluten can be found in wheat, rye, barley and any foods made with these grains. Gluten sensitivity can cause weight gain as well as digestive problems, fatigue, and inflammation to name a few. Being sensitive to gluten can cause a hormonal imbalance and disrupt the thyroid function. When you stop eating what your body is sensitive to, it can result in healthy weight loss. This happens because the body tends to hold water to protect itself from something it is sensitive to. When the offensive food is taken out of the diet, the water goes with it.

The Paleo diet eliminates grains from your diet. This alone can cause a decrease in weight if you have gluten intolerance. If you suspect that you might be sensitive to gluten, research non-grain foods that have hidden gluten in them in order to make sure that you are excluding gluten entirely from your diet. Though gluten is mostly found in grains it can surprisingly be found in non-grain foods as well.

Diabetes

The Paleo diet fights diabetes by addressing the root of the problem: diet and lifestyle that don't support the body's needs. Because the Paleo diet eliminates refined sugars, processed foods and carbohydrates, and replaces them with good fats and protein, the body stays balanced and avoids triggered glucose spikes that lead to insulin resistance.

As well as eating foods that support a healthy body, the Paleo lifestyle also stresses regular physical activity and an adequate amount of sleep. These are both necessary in controlling diabetes.

Clinical studies have proven that the Paleo diet is an effective way to control diabetes. In fact, the Paleo diet is even more effective at controlling diabetes than the popular Mediterranean diet. Diabetics can tailor the Paleo diet to suit their specific needs, making it an even more effective, individualized plan for better health.

Acne

Recent studies show the connection between acne and a person's diet. The Paleo diet works to prevent the different stages of acne development. Because a Paleo diet has a low glycemic load compared to a typical western diet, it reduces the production of insulin. Evidence has shown that a hormonal imbalance caused by diet-induced hyper insulin promotes unregulated tissue growth and androgen-mediated sebum excretion leading to acne.

Dairy is one of the dietary culprits that are said to cause acne. Milk and milk products are capable of increasing insulin levels and IGF-1. These are both stimulators that cause acne. These two hormones increase the production of sebum; a fat, and carotene; a protein within hair follicles. This causes a build up of sebum and carotene in hair follicles that can cause blockages. This can result in increased acne symptoms.

Just as a note, whey protein is a particularly strong stimulator of the hormones insulin and IGF-1. Surprisingly, it can be worse for acne than milk.

Along with eliminating dairy, the Paleo diet also excludes grains which are thought to play a role in causing acne as well.

The most important thing that you should eliminate from your diet if you suffer from acne is sugar. Consuming sugar, particularly sugar with higher fructose levels can lead to problems with your body's response to insulin. It causes your body to pump out too much sugar which causes hormone changes. This increases acne symptoms.

The Paleo diet also promotes a dietary lifestyle that is rich in nutrients such as omega 3 and EPA. These nutrients can reduce inflammation and redness associated with acne.

Paleo for men

According to researchers, men find it difficult to metabolize their carbohydrates which leads to obesity, chronic illness, lung problems and even cancer. The Paleo diet does not only fight obesity but also helps men tone their body for optimal physical strength and lean muscles. By decreasing the consumption of food that is high in its glycemic load and replacing it with nutrient-dense food, weight management becomes easier. The high levels of protein in the diet help replenish the muscles after a rigorous workout.

Having an optimal physique increases longevity and keeps the body strong and alive. Prostate cancer can also be avoided by cutting fatty meat and dairy products from your diet.

Paleo for women

Women often choose to get on a Paleo diet to gain optimal physical performance and to lose excess body fat. The diet helps stabilize blood sugar and decrease the overall consumption of carbohydrates causing the female body to shed pounds. It is important to remember though that while women are on the Paleo diet, they should decrease their fruit and fat intake. Eating healthy fat from nuts or those from olive oil is essential to a healthy diet but too much can cause unwanted weight gain.

Pregnant women can benefit from the Paleo diet. Omega-3 in the form of DHA is essential in the development of the growing baby. A diet that is high in fruits and vegetables like the Paleo diet, provides women with the adequate dose of folate and minerals to reduce the chances of the baby having neural tube defects.

Women who have health conditions related to the reproductive organs or menstrual cycle can also benefit from a Palaeolithic diet. PCOS or polycystic ovarian syndrome causes symptoms like long menstruation periods, no menstruation period, facial hair, baldness, acne and ovarian cysts. The Paleo diet can combat these symptoms by eliminating grains.

The main concern that women have with the Paleo diet is that it might cause osteoporosis in the future because it does not allow the consumption of dairy products. Plant-based food can provide all the essential calcium needed by the body. In fact, plant-based calcium can be absorbed better than dairy-based calcium. Women only need to eat a strict Paleo diet consisting of dark leafy green vegetables for calcium and vitamin D. This will increase health, vitality and promote healthy bones throughout the menopausal stage.

Paleo for kids

A baby raised on a Paleo diet often relies on breast milk as the source of nutrition from birth to age one. At the age of one, generally all food that is consumed by adults can be fed to the child. Some Paleo parents even give bones to their babies to chew on for teething.

Slightly mash food like cooked meat or potatoes for young children. Other foods like vegetables should be chopped in smaller pieces for easy swallowing. Do not overcook the food in order to retain as much of the nutrients as possible. Buy organic food to minimize the toxins entering the child's body. Most mega-farms use antibiotics, hormones and herbicides that can be transferred to their crops, so organic is always the best way to go.

Many enthusiasts follow a baby-led weaning technique where the baby chooses what, when and how much to eat. Simply offer the baby a variety of choices at each meal like meat, vegetables and a limited quantity of fruit, and then allow the baby to feed themselves.

Some babies refuse to drink breast milk after tasting solid food while some reject solid food and opt for breast milk. Every child is different, allow the child to have their own freedom in weaning.

Paleo for older generations

Most people believe that because early cavemen lived a short and brutal life their diet must have been poor and ineffective. Truth is, cavemen usually died because of trauma and accidents and not because of a poor diet. Hunter-gatherer societies that exist today have an abundance of people older than 60 who are much healthier than their western counterparts.

According to the research done by ARPF, the perfect diet to prevent Alzheimer's disease is one that is rich in healthy fats, complex carbohydrates and lean proteins. The Paleo diet falls in line with the anti-Alzheimer diet which advocates the consumption of healthy fat, lean proteins and complex carbohydrates.

Rheumatoid arthritis, an inflammatory disease which is most common in middle-aged people, can affect the joints, skin and lungs. By increasing the intake of omega 3 fatty acids and by reducing the intake of omega-6 fatty acids, there can be a decrease in the negative effects of arthritis in the body.

The Paleo diet is known for its anti-inflammatory benefits and for its ability to fight against autoimmune diseases.

Chapter 4

How Does the Paleo Diet Compare?

Paleo vs. Vegan

The primary difference between the Paleo and Vegan diet is the consumption of meat. Vegans only eat plant-based food and reject animal products while the Paleo diet focuses on what our early ancestors ate. The problem with a vegan diet is that it includes too much processed food including flour and sweeteners. Even potato chips are considered vegan as long as they are 'plant-based'. A vegan can also be susceptible to diabetes even by only eating fruits and grains.

Paleo vs. The Zone Diet

The Paleo diet involves an unweighed and unmeasured diet of quality food while the Zone diet follows a specific ratio of macronutrients that is needed by the body for optimum performance. The Zone diet uses a ratio of 40% carbohydrates, 30% protein and 30% fat. The proponents of this diet believe that by using this ratio, the release of insulin and glucagon will be controlled, thus decreasing the risk of heart ailments. However, for someone who is not big on measuring everything they eat, the Paleo diet proves to be more beneficial.

Paleo vs. The Mediterranean Diet

The Mediterranean diet consists of a high intake of olive oil, nuts and fruits as well as vegetables and cereals while lowering the intake of animal products. The main problem with the Mediterranean diet is that there is rarely any significant weight loss acquired from it. Replacing saturated fat with olive oil simply transfers one type of fat to another. There is also research that proves that the Paleo diet is more effective than the Mediterranean diet in lowering sugar levels for people with type 2 Diabetes.

Paleo vs. The Atkins Diet

The Paleo diet and the Atkins diet are both considered low carbohydrate diets but there are many differences between the two. The Atkins diet does not specify the source of meat that should be eaten on their diet. It could be factory farmed, corn-fed or antibiotic laced. The diet is only specific about eating a lot of protein and fat with little carbohydrates. The Paleo diet on the other hand, clearly states the importance of eating wild and grass fed meats for their high nutrient content. The Atkins diet also promotes using oil such as sunflower, grape seed or vegetable oil raw or for cooking. These oils are rich in omega 6 fatty acids that promote inflammation. The Atkins diet also allows the use of artificial sweeteners which the Paleo diet advocates against.

Chapter 5

How the Paleo Diet is Your Body's Best Friend

The Paleo Diet is without question the best "all natural" diet you can choose. It exclusively promotes eating the way our ancestors did and it doesn't add anything artificial or processed to the mix as some diets do.

The unadulterated foods that our ancestors ate complimented the intricate workings of the human body and therefore enhanced its performance. Because the foods were "clean" and natural, the body could easily recognize them and efficiently convert them into energy.

Nowadays, about 25% of people in North America unknowingly suffer from metabolic syndrome (an energy utilization and storage disorder) because their bodies are unable to turn food into usable energy.

What you'll find after switching to the Paleo Diet is that you'll feel a lot better. Your energy will increase and you'll feel more connected and in tune with your body's nutritional needs.

When you give your body what it wants it will reward you with great health and vitality.

Outlined below are the ways in which the Paleo diet works with the human body to create optimal health. It truly is your body's best friend!

A healthier brain

Omega 3 fatty acids are essential fatty acids that are a necessary part of our diet. The human body can't make omega 3 fatty acids so it has to get them from food. Omega 3's, as they are commonly called, can be found in salmon, halibut, tuna and other seafood. Algae, various plants and nut oils also contain omega 3's.

Though brain health is not the only benefit of omega 3's, the brain tends to have highly concentrated omega 3 fatty acids that are associated with cognitive and behavioral function.

The average North American diet is lacking in omega 3 fatty acids. Paleolithic eating highly advocates getting our protein and fat from cold water fish, particularly wild salmon. Salmon fat is jam-packed with healthy omega 3's that contain DHA that support brain function and development.

Healthier cells

Our cells function at their best when there is a healthy balance of saturated and unsaturated fat in the body. Why? Because cells are made from both saturated and unsaturated fat. The balance of these two fats in the cells allow them to efficiently send messages in and out.

In modern society there is a significant imbalance in these two fats. Saturated fats tend to be consumed much more than unsaturated fats therefore throwing off this necessary balance and taking a toll on our cells.

Some diets limit one or the other kind of fat but the Paleo diet provides an ideal balance of both saturated and unsaturated fat. This allows our cells to maintain good health and function at their best.

Digestive health benefits

Foods that have been processed and altered from their natural state are much more difficult for the body to digest. Imagine the body and nature as being one. Next, imagine natural foods on earth as specifically being designed to nurture and nourish the body.

It makes sense then that eating from the earth will serve the body best. This isn't difficult to understand, it's just about getting back to the basics.

The Paleo diet suggests eating foods that your body has grown accustom to digesting best over thousands of years. Your body has no problem recognizing and digesting an apple, a berry or grass-fed meat. That's why the Paleo diet can keep your digestive health in check.

Reduced inflammation

Inflammation can wreak havoc on the body. In fact, research has suggested that inflammation is a key contributor for many life-threatening diseases. Much of the food on the Paleo diet is anti-inflammatory therefore it reduces your risk of developing inflammatory based diseases.

Increased muscle

Let's face it; you eat a lot of meat on the Paleo diet. This is a good thing because meat is an excellent source of protein. Protein is necessary in order to build brand new cells that we commonly recognize as muscle.

Whenever you've got more muscle on your body than fat, your metabolism automatically works better. This happens because muscles require energy to move. When your muscles are more prominent, your energy will be directed to muscle cells instead of fat cells. This will in turn help you lose fat.

Losing fat is a good thing since many diseases occur as a result of being overweight.

Reduces allergies

Grains and dairy are known to be allergens in certain societies. The Paleo diet recognizes this and recommends removing both for a minimum of one month in order to cleanse your system.

This gives your body a chance to 're-group' and get things back in order in case it is secretly harboring a dislike for grains or dairy. As your body undergoes a cleansing from these foods you will become more sensitive to knowing whether or not these foods were silently causing fatigue or ill feelings. If so, you can make the necessary adjustments that will allow you to function at your best.

Chapter 6

Seven Day Meal Plan and Recipes

Choosing to create Paleo meals and stick to a Paleo diet involves planning. In starting a Paleo diet, be patient because there will be a lot of trial and error involved in finding recipes that suit your budget and taste.

Be open to trying new foods and new spices and avoid being a slave to habit by only eating foods that you know you like or are most used to. Be adventurous and you might find something you really love!

Here are some delicious Paleo recipes and a seven day meal plan.

Monday

Breakfast

Sweet Potato and Onion Tortilla Espanola

1 sweet potato, thinly sliced

¼ onion, sliced

½ cup coconut oil

6 eggs, whisked

Salt and pepper

Heat the coconut oil in a skillet over medium-low heat then add the thinly sliced sweet potato. Brown on both sides. Add the sliced onions and cook until they are opaque. Pour in the whisked eggs and gently mix them with the potato and onions. Set on low heat and allow the eggs to cook for 5 more minutes. Season to taste. Serve.

Lunch

Fancy Chicken Salad

2 chicken breasts, diced

1 English cucumber, cut into thin slices

1 cup seedless grapes, halved

½ cup Paleo mayonnaise (see recipe below)

¼ cup chopped walnuts

2 finely chopped celery stalks

Combine chicken, celery, walnuts and Paleo mayonnaise in a medium sized bowl. Assemble the thinly sliced cucumber on a serving plate then top with the chicken mixture. Sprinkle with sliced grapes and serve.

Paleo mayonnaise:

1 large egg

1 ½ tbsp lemon juice

½ tsp dry mustard

½ cup extra virgin olive oil

½ cup avocado oil

¼ tsp ground white pepper

In a food processor combine the egg, lemon juice and dry mustard. Blend until frothy. With the food processor running, drizzle in the olive oil and avocado oil slowly until smooth and creamy. Season with white pepper. Put the mayonnaise in a sealed container and refrigerate.

Snack

Apple Cinnamon Muffins

Dry ingredients:

¼ cup coconut flour

¼ cup almond flour

¼ tsp baking soda

1 ½ tsp cinnamon

½ tsp sea salt

Wet ingredients:

5 eggs

2 green apples

¼ cup maple syrup

½ cup coconut milk

¼ cup coconut oil

Preheat the oven to 350 degrees. Lightly grease 12 muffin tins.

Combine all the dry ingredients in a small bowl. Mix together all the wet ingredients except the apples and coconut oil in a large bowl. Gradually blend the dry ingredients into the wet ingredients then stir in the apples and melted coconut oil. Let the mixture sit for 10 minutes before spooning it into the muffin tin. Bake for 20 minutes and allow the muffins to cool before removing.

Dinner

Stir-Fried Beef and Noodles

4 cups spaghetti (grain free, Paleo pasta or Kelp noodles)

1 lb sirloin or flank steak, sliced into strips

1 tbsp coconut oil

¼ cup coconut aminos

1-2 stalks celery

½ cup zucchini

1 medium yellow onion

Raw honey

2 tbsp of almonds

In a small bowl, mix together the coconut aminos and raw honey. Set aside. Heat coconut oil in a skillet and add the vegetables. Sauté for 3 minutes. Add the steak. Heat through. Reduce the heat then add the aminos/honey mixture. Toss in the spaghetti and sprinkle with almonds.

Tuesday

Breakfast

Paleo Coffee Cake Banana Bread

3 ripe bananas, mashed

¼ cup maple syrup

1 tsp vanilla extract

3 eggs

½ cup almond butter (or other nut/seed butter)

¼ cup coconut flour

½ tsp baking soda

½ tsp baking powder

1 tsp cinnamon

Dash of salt

For the toppings:

¼ cup grass fed butter, at room temperature (or coconut oil)

2 tbsp coconut sugar

2 tbsp almond flour

1 tsp cinnamon

¼ cup pecans, crushed

Preheat the oven to 350 degrees. Grease an 8.5 x 4.5 baking dish with oil and line the middle of the dish with parchment paper. Mix the first four ingredients together in a large bowl (bananas, maple syrup, vanilla extract, eggs). Add the remaining five ingredients to the bowl and mix (coconut flour, baking soda, baking powder, cinnamon and salt). Pour the batter into the baking dish.

In a small bowl combine the five topping ingredients and mix them together with your hands. Chunk the topping all over the top of the bread mixture. Place in oven and bake for 50 minutes. Remove from oven and place the bread on a cooling rack. Let it rest there for 10 minutes. Cut and serve.

Lunch

Roasted Veggies

2 heads broccoli florets

1 cauliflower

2 sweet potatoes

15 Brussels sprouts

2-3 beets

Garlic

Extra virgin olive oil

Salt and pepper to taste

Place all the vegetables on a greased baking sheet and sprinkle with olive oil. Season with salt and pepper. Place the pan in the oven and roast for 50 minutes.

<u>Snack</u>

Raw Apple with Caramel Almond Butter

1 apple

1 tsp almond butter

Core the apple then slice it into thin pieces. Layer each slice with one teaspoon of almond butter and enjoy!

Dinner

Lettuce Taco

Taco seasoning, to taste

2 tbsp cumin

1-1/2 tbsp chilli powder

1 tbsp garlic powder

1 tbsp onion powder

2 tsp smoked paprika

2 tsp salt

1 lb extra lean ground beef

1 head iceberg lettuce, thinly sliced

2 tbsp extra virgin olive oil

Heat olive oil in a skillet. Add the ground beef and brown on low heat. Mix all the remaining ingredients together in a bowl.

Add the contents of the bowl to the beef. Wrap the beef in the lettuce. Serve.

Wednesday

Breakfast

Paleo Style Banana Pancakes

1 egg

1 banana

Sea salt

1 tbsp cinnamon

1 tbsp almond flour

Fresh strawberries, blueberries and/or blackberries

Pure honey or maple syrup

4 tbsp extra virgin olive oil

Heat the oil in a skillet on medium-low heat. In a bowl, mash the bananas with a fork. Add the egg to the bowl and blend well. Add the cinnamon and a dash of sea salt. With a spoon or ice cream scoop, pour enough pancake batter onto the pan to make a small pancake. Continue to create as many pancakes as you can with the batter. Allow the pancakes to brown lightly on the edges before flipping. When both sides have been lightly browned, remove from pan. Top with fresh strawberries blueberries and/or blackberries. Drizzle with honey or maple syrup. Serve.

Lunch

Stir-Fried Noodles with Steak and Mushrooms

1 package kelp noodles

1 tsp coconut oil

4 scallions

2/3 pound sirloin steak, thinly sliced

2 cups mushrooms

Garlic, to taste

6 ounces baby spinach

2 tbsp vinegar

2 tbsp lime juice

3 tsp coconut aminos

1 tbsp ginger

2 tsp sriracha

1 tsp dark sesame seeds

Melt the oil in a large skillet. Sauté the onions and steak then add mushrooms and garlic. Add the baby spinach and stir until the greens wilt. Combine vinegar, lime juice, coconut aminos, ginger and sriracha in a small bowl then add to the skillet. Cook for 30 seconds and add the kelp noodles. Cook through. Sprinkle with the sesame seeds. Serve.

<u>Snack</u>

Cinnamon Granola

1 cup raw almonds

½ cup shredded coconut

½ cup chopped walnuts

½ cup pure maple syrup

1 tsp cinnamon

Sea salt to taste

Pre-heat the oven to 350 degrees. Mix all the nuts in a bowl then add the maple syrup and cinnamon. Spread the mixture on a baking sheet and sprinkle with salt. Bake for 15 minutes.

<u>Dinner</u>

Stuffed Bell Peppers

2 red bell peppers

1 pound ground beef

2 garlic cloves

½ medium yellow onion

1 can diced tomatoes

1 zucchini, chopped

2 eggs

Guacamole

Salad or veggies of choice

Brown the ground beef in a skillet. Add onion and garlic. Cook for 4 minutes then add the zucchini. Cook for another 3 minutes. Remove from heat then add the tomatoes and eggs. Cut off the top of the pepper and set aside. Scoop out the seeds and spoon the meat mixture into the pepper. Place the top of the pepper back on. Fill a casserole dish with water just enough to cover about an inch of the bottom of each pepper. Place the peppers upright in the water. Bake for 30 minutes until the peppers are lightly brown. Top with guacamole.

Thursday

Breakfast

Avocado and Bacon Omelet

4 bacon slices

1 avocado

2 red onions

Hot sauce

4 eggs

Cilantro, minced

Cook the bacon until crisp. Slice the avocado in half and scoop the flesh into a bowl then mash. Add onion and cilantro to the avocado. Cut the bacon in small pieces and add to the avocado mixture. Pour the avocado mixture onto a pan then add the eggs to make omelettes.

Lunch

Menemen

1 garlic clove, minced

¼ diced red onion

1 medium tomato

½ cup yellow bell pepper

1 tbsp extra virgin olive oil

¼ tsp ground cumin

¼ tsp black pepper

¼ tsp salt

3 eggs

¼ tsp turmeric

1 tbsp minced fresh parsley

Sauté the red onion, pepper, and tomato in the olive oil. Add the garlic and spices. Stir until vegetables soften. Whisk eggs in a dish. When the vegetables have softened and created a sauce, add the eggs and scramble until the mixture has lightly set. Sprinkle with parsley. Serve.

Snack

Cauliflower Popcorn

1 head of cauliflower

4 tbsp extra virgin olive oil

Sea salt

Pre-heat oven to 400 degrees. Trim the head of cauliflower and cut it into tiny pieces. Combine olive oil and salt into a bowl then add cauliflower. Roast for an hour until most pieces are golden brown. Serve.

Dinner

Liver and Onions with Bacon

2 lbs beef liver, sliced

1 large yellow onion

4 garlic cloves, crushed

6 slices of bacon

1 cup of mushrooms

Salt

Pepper

Crisp the bacon in a skillet. Add onions, garlic and mushrooms. Cook through. Remove the bacon mixture from the skillet and keep warm. Add beef liver to the skillet and cook through for about 10 minutes. When the liver has been seared on both sides, top it with the onion, garlic, mushrooms and bacon. Season with salt and pepper. Serve.

Friday

Breakfast

Cinnamon-Honey Paleonola

2 cups shredded coconut meat

1 cup flaxseed meal

1 tsp ground cinnamon

1/3 cup honey

½ tsp salt

½ cup water

¼ cup sesame seeds

½ cup coconut oil, melted

½ cup sliced almonds

½ cup shelled pumpkin seeds

½ cup sunflower seeds

2 cups chopped pecans

½ cup chopped walnuts

Preheat the oven to 250 degrees. In a medium bowl combine the flax meal, coconut meat, cinnamon, sesame seeds and salt. Stir. In a separate bowl, mix water, coconut oil and honey together. Pour the water mixture over the dry ingredients. Whisk until everything is damp.

Line an 11x13 inch roasting pan with non-stick foil. Pour the mixture into the pan. Press it into an even layer and bake for 1 hour. Cut into 1 inch squares. Scoop up those squares and stir them around in the pan. They'll crumble and you can cut larger pieces into ½ pieces.

Measure and stir in the nuts and seeds. Put the pan back in the oven for 20 minutes. After 20 minutes stir everything again and put the pan back in the oven. Repeat a few more times until the nuts and seeds have been toasted to your liking. Remove from oven, cool and store in a tightly lidded container.

Lunch

Egg Salad

½ diced bell pepper

2 celery stalks, chopped

2 tbsp fresh parsley chopped

4 scallions, chopped

6 hard-boiled eggs, chopped

1 tbsp brown mustard

Paleo mayonnaise, to taste (find recipe under Monday lunch)

Salt and pepper

In a bowl stir together all the vegetables and eggs. Stir in the mustard and Paleo mayonnaise. Sprinkle with salt and pepper. Serve.

Snack

Bacon and Guacamole Sandwich

4 strips of thick cut bacon

1 avocado

1 lime

Salt

Wrap the bacon between sheets of paper towel and heat in the microwave. Mash up the flesh of half the avocado. Dice the other half. Mix the two halves together. Add a few squirts of lime juice. Add sea salt. Sandwich the avocado between two pieces of bacon strips and serve.

Dinner

Chicken Fajitas

3 lbs chicken breast, thinly sliced

3 onions, sliced

3 red bell peppers

2 tbsp of chilli powder, cumin and oregano

6 garlic cloves, chopped

2 tbsp coriander

5 lemons, juiced

Butter lettuce

4 tbsp coconut oil

Salsa

Guacamole

In a bowl, mix the chicken, onions, red bell peppers, spices, lemon juice and garlic together. Marinate in fridge for 4 hours. After 4 hours, heat a skillet on medium heat. Add the marinated chicken and cook through. Scoop chicken into butter lettuce leaves and top with salsa and guacamole.

Saturday

Breakfast

Zucchini Pancakes

1 medium zucchini

1 scallion, chopped

1 egg

Sea salt

Pepper

2 tbsp extra virgin olive oil

Heat the oil in a skillet on medium-low heat. Grate zucchini into a bowl. Add scallion. Crack the egg into the bowl, season with salt and pepper and mix well. Pour the egg mixture onto the pan into three pancake shapes and fry until brown on each side. Serve.

Lunch

Spinach, Mushroom and Cherry Stir-Fry

1 tsp butter

2 tbsp extra virgin olive oil

½ red onion, sliced

¾ cup cherry tomatoes, halved

6 button mushrooms, sliced

3 large handfuls torn spinach leaves

1 garlic clove, finely chopped

½ tsp lemon rind

2/3 tsp sea salt

Pepper

Nutmeg

1 lemon

Heat butter in frying pan and sauté mushrooms. Remove and keep warm. In the same pan, sauté the onions. Add tomatoes, lemon rind and garlic. Season with salt, pepper and nutmeg. Cook for 3 minutes. Add spinach and stir. Drizzle with lemon juice and season with salt to taste. Serve with eggs.

Snack

Roasted Sweet Potato

1 small cubed sweet potato

½ onion, chopped

¼ tsp cayenne pepper

½ green bell pepper

¼ cup grape tomatoes

1 tbsp cilantro

1 egg

Salt and pepper

Cook potatoes and onions in olive oil. Add cayenne pepper and salt, cover for 5 minutes until softened. Add all the ingredients except the egg. Make an impression in the middle of the mixture and crack the egg into the hole. Cook for 3 minutes then garnish with cilantro. Season with salt and pepper.

Dinner

Baked Salmon with Roasted Beets and Asparagus

4 salmon fillets

4 tbsp coconut oil

4 tsp chopped dill

4 red beets in cubes

16 fresh asparagus spears

Salt and pepper

Preheat the oven to 450 degrees. Lay 4 asparagus spears on a sheet of tin foil. The tin foil will create a packet. On top of the asparagus spears arrange 4 beets then place the salmon fillet on top of the 4 beet cubes. Add 1 tbsp of oil, salt, pepper and dill. Fold the foil to make a packet and bake in the oven for 10 minutes for each thickness of the fish. Approx 30 minutes.

Sunday

Breakfast

Asian Pepper Shrimp

1 ½ lbs shrimp, raw, peeled, tail on

3 tbsp coconut oil

4 cloves of garlic

1 tbsp coconut aminos

1 tbsp fish sauce

¼ cup cilantro

1 tsp black pepper

Melt coconut oil. Sauté the garlic for 2 minutes then add shrimp and sauté for 5 minutes. Stir in the coconut aminos, pepper and fish sauce. Sauté further. Plate the shrimp and pour the remaining liquid in the pan on top of the shrimp. Top with a tablespoon of cilantro.

Lunch

Crunchy chicken

4 chicken legs

1 tsp curry powder

½ cup almond meal

1 tsp cayenne pepper

1 tsp dry mustard

4 tbsp extra virgin olive oil

Combine almond meal with seasonings. Rub the chicken with olive oil then roll in the almond meal mixture. Roast for an hour until the coating is crunchy. Serve.

Snack

Kale Chips

1 bunch kale

¼ tsp sea salt

1 tsp olive oil

Wash the kale and remove tough stems. Cut the kale into strips and place on baking sheet. Drizzle with salt and olive oil then toss the kale to coat. Bake for 15 minutes until the kale is crispy. Serve.

Dinner

White Wine and Garlic mussels

4 lbs fresh mussels

2 cups white wine

2 onions, chopped

5 garlic cloves, chopped

6 tbsp butter (ghee)

1/3 cup fresh basil

In a pot, combine the white wine, garlic and onions and bring to a boil. Lower heat and simmer for about 5 minutes. Add in the mussels' then cover. Bring to a boil. When the mussels open add the fresh basil and butter then remove from heat. Serve with wine, butter sauce and garlic.

Chapter 7
Tips for Sticking with the Paleo Diet

There can be many challenges that you encounter while on the Paleo diet. Here are some tips to stay on track.

Paleo while eating out

When dining out, choose a source of protein as well as healthy fats along with vegetables. Get lettuce wraps instead of burgers. Some of the best restaurants that support the Paleo diet are Mongolian barbeques. Plus they usually allow their customers to choose their own meats and oils.

Paleo on a budget

Buy foods that are in season so as to take advantage of low prices and sales. Focus on buying cheaper produce with more nutrients. You can also consider planting a garden in order to grow your own organic vegetables and herbs.

Paleo while travelling

Take a cooler with you and stash it with healthy snacks like carrot sticks, apples, bananas and other transportable foods. Some Paleo dieters use the travel time to fast. With a little creativity, you can stick to your Paleo diet while on the road. Some planning will be necessary but being organized will make your trip enjoyable, relaxing and healthy.

Other books by Gina Crawford

Mediterranean Diet for Beginners

Mediterranean Diet Cookbook

DASH Diet for Beginners

DASH Diet Cookbook

The 5:2 Diet for Beginners

5:2 Diet 30 Minute Recipes

Sugar Detox for Beginners

Sugar Free Recipes

Available on Amazon

Conclusion

Congratulations on finishing the book!

I pour my heart into every book and make every effort to help you achieve your diet and health goals.

I hope this book gave you all the necessary information you needed to understand the Paleo diet better and apply it to your life to achieve optimum health.

About Gina Crawford

Understanding what it takes to live a healthy lifestyle, eat right, achieve your goal weight and love your life shouldn't be complicated. Your time is valuable and the last thing you need is to tackle a 300 page book on how to get your health, weight and life on track. If you're like most people, you just want the facts in bite-sized, easy to understand pieces that you can apply to your life TODAY!

My name is Gina Crawford. I am a health and "all things natural" enthusiast, author, mother and wife. Years ago I was overweight, exhausted, unhappy and desperately aching for a better life. One day, gruelingly tired of my situation, I started researching everything I could on health and transforming my life. Often I felt overwhelmed by the amount of information and the changes I had to make, but I persevered and managed to turn my life around one book and one bite at a time.

Now I'm determined to share what I've learned in an easy, non-overwhelming, "no fluff, no filler, straight to the point" kind of way that will allow others to achieve maximum results in a short amount of time.

I am passionate about every book I write and my goal with each book is to make it simple and concise yet power-packed with the necessary information you need to transform your life. I have learned first-hand the incredible value of healing ourselves with natural organic foods, natural remedies, exercise and a positive mindset.

When I'm not writing, I love spending time with my family, cooking, walking, biking and reading.

Thank you for purchasing my book. My hope is that it will help you live a healthier, better, more passionate, alive life!

Happy reading!

Gina